I0791097

Natural Virus Protection

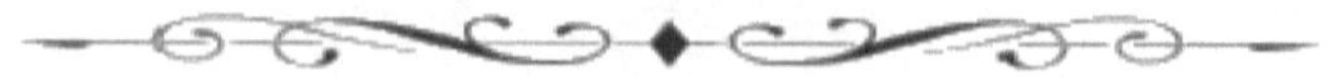

Companion books linked to "Natural Virus Protection"
are recommended reading for more detailed information.

Pure, White and Deadly, by John Yudkin
How sugar is killing us and what we can do to stop it.
In his 1972 book, Dr. John Yudkin, a United Kingdom nutritionist, conducted detailed research into the deleterious effects of sugar. His studies showed that sugar and other refined carbohydrates like sugar-sweetened beverages, pastries, white bread, white pasta, white rice and others were more dangerous even than fat intake for adverse effects on the human body and could weaken natural immunities to disease and other disorders.

Vermont Folk Medicine by Dr. D.C. Jarvis
A famous doctor's 1958 guide to folk medicine practices on the nature of Honey and Apple Cider Vinegar to improve your overall health. Dr. Jarvis' purpose is to bring knowledge and understanding of the capability and uses of folk medicine for improving natural body immunity to be free of physical impairment and weakness from disease and virus infections.

These two doctor's prophetic understanding of the natural immunity found in the human body show how humans are easily led through advertising to eat foods for taste rather than for health. However you do not have to give up your favorite foods if you follow the recommendations in this book to limit or to add some simple additives to return to good health and natural immunity to diseases.

Natural Virus Protection

Improving your natural Immunity to the 2020 Coronavirus (COVID-19)

by Marlys J. Waters, editor

Power of the Pen Publishing
Nemaha, Iowa

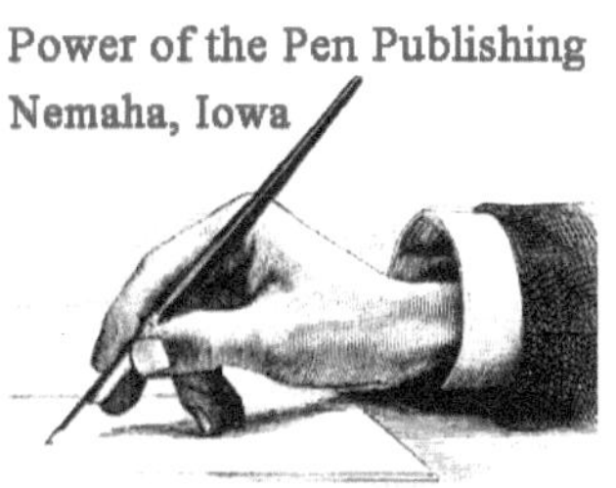

ISBN-13: 978-1-67800-020-2

Published by:
Power of the Pen Publishing
PO Box 5
Nemaha, IA 50567

Table of Contents

Preface by Marlys J. Waters

I believe it is important in 2020 to get some out-of-print "do-it-yourself" health books back into circulation for the modern times when we expect physicians to cure everything with a pill, an injection, or an operation.

Some modern medications may cure one ailment but cause something worse. That is why I am republishing books from the past that helped maintain our health when more studies were being done on humans brave enough to try different foods, lifestyles, and exercise rather than current pharmaceutical labs that only work at the molecular level with pills.

Don't get me wrong, the cure for polio, measles, suppression of HIV/AIDS, syphilis, bubonic plague and other scourges of the past have been laid to rest by medical science.

Also included are discussions of the various treatments for disease, as well as an index and an appendix of food value charts.

There are now new health disorders that are creeping in which don't seem to respond to previous treatments for viruses, some bacteria, germs, microbes, and other pathogens. Autism is one recent controversial disorder that is still being studied and is not discussed in this book.

With modern genetic testing on the source of our food products, it is always safe to go back to the olden days when you raised your own garden produce without the use of genetically modified seeds and fertilizers that may no longer host the trace vitamins and minerals that are so important to our health.

In other words, don't expect the doctor to cure all your sickness with a pill, a shot, or surgery. Your very health may start at home with a book. Many great minds left behind their knowledge in the form of books. Don't be hesitant to pick up a dusty copy published many years earlier. Brilliant minds may have already invented home cures for other physical disorders.

One further warning: Don't believe everything you hear and read, trust your intuition. There are also some quacks that have written books which can ruin your health.

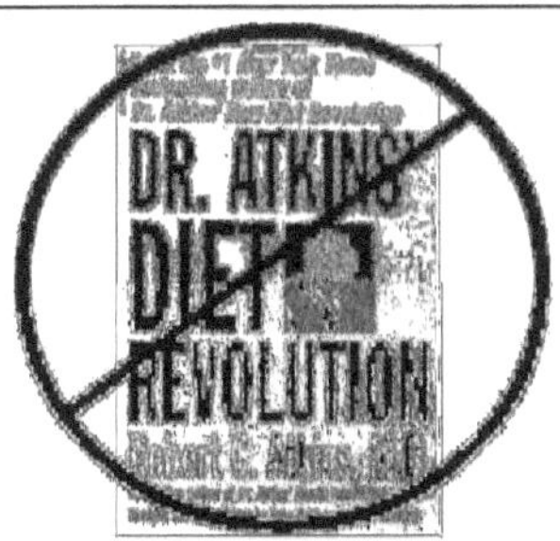

DO NOT subscribe to the theory of Dr. Robert Atkins book: *"Dr. Atkin's Diet Revolution"*. He was the diet doctor who popularized the notion that dieters could eat fat and high protein and lose weight. He died on April 17, 2003, at the age 72. He had a history of heart attack and congestive heart failure. He weighed 258 pounds at his death.

While his book was a best-seller, a lot of people ended up with high blood pressure that could damage the heart, cause strokes, and other side affects. I tried the diet and lost a little weight but was having my blood pressure checked monthly when I donated blood at a blood center. Fortunately the increasing and dangerous high blood pressure was noted and I realized it was that high-protein/fat diet which caused it. Others were also reporting in the media the same dangerous side affects.

Be your own guinea pig with your health but pay attention to your vital signs. Keep track of your results. Discontinue anything you may read in any book that makes you feel worse.

I recommend that people read books that teach you something about health, relationships, or self-betterment. You'll be a better person for it and might even live longer and healthier.

The comments in this preface are mine and I take responsibility for any misinformation found on these two pages.

You are on your own for the balance of the book that was compiled from research by physicians and scientists who tested and analyzed humans resulting in books to enlighten the reader.
~ Marlys J. Waters

The 2020 Coronavirus - COVID-19

The latest wide spread virus infection in the northern hemisphere called the **Coronavirus or COVID-19**, is spreading panic across several continents.

This is one (of many) news updates on March 4, 2020:

- California reported its first death from COVID-19, in an elderly adult with underlying health conditions, the Sacramento Bee reported. The resident of Placer County had taken a cruise from San Francisco to Mexico Feb. 11 to Feb. 21 and was potentially exposed while abroad.

- Italy's government announced Wednesday all schools and universities in the country will be closed from March 5 to March 15, as the country now has more than 2,500 cases and 79 deaths linked to the coronavirus, CNBC reported.

- Los Angeles County reported six new cases of the novel coronavirus on Wednesday (March 4). All of the cases are linked with an "assumed known exposure," such as a history of travel, exposure to a traveler or close contact with a known case, officials said. The county declared a local health emergency to better prepare for and respond to the virus.

- The global mortality rate for COVID-19 is 3.4%, WHO said on March 2. This virus causes more severe illness than the flu, but doesn't spread as efficiently, <u>the director-general said</u>.

- The Olympic Games, scheduled for this summer in Tokyo, will likely continue as planned but there's a chance it <u>could be postponed</u> until later this year amid the coronavirus outbreak.

- Washington state reported three more deaths from the coronavirus on Tuesday.

- FDA announces 1 million coronavirus tests should be available by end of week.

5

- There are now at least 128 confirmed cases in the U.S., with 31 of those in Washington state, which also has the first related deaths (nine).
- 94,250 confirmed coronavirus cases worldwide, with more cases popping up outside China than inside.
- 3,214 deaths have been linked to the virus. Deaths worldwide exceed those from SARS. And 51,026 individuals have recovered from COVID-19.
- Cases of coronavirus in South Korea have skyrocketed to 5,621, where about 60% of the cases are somehow linked to members of a secret religious sect.

Is there a reason to panic? Not if you understand that this is just one more of many viruses that threaten the northern hemisphere every winter.

So should we stop mixing with other people, close all the schools, churches, quit traveling, lock up all small businesses? NO! Humans who are healthy will not become infected with the virus if they know how to keep their system healthy. A healthy human body fights daily against invading germs, virus, common colds and much more.

Our eating habits are what are lowering our resistance to infections and other health disorders. Surprisingly the solution is very simple and has been around for years. Read on. . .

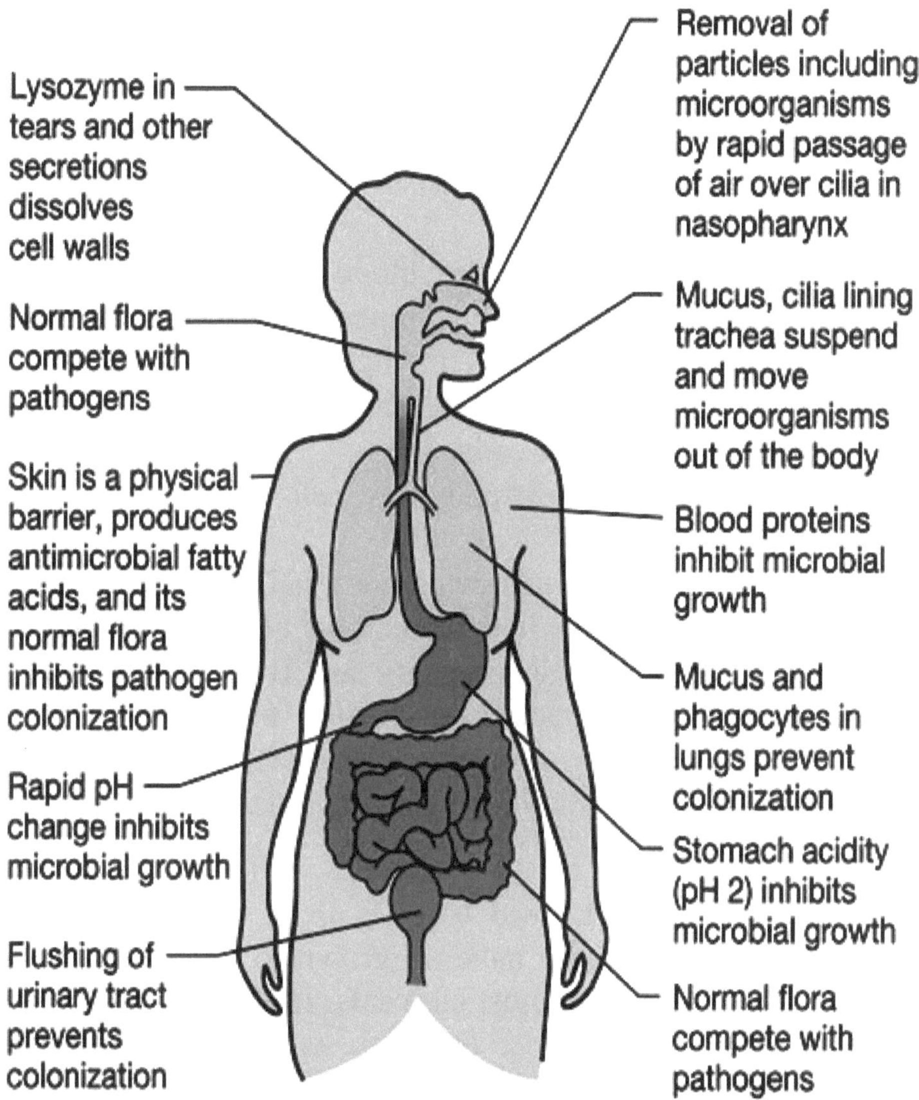

So if the human body has all this natural immunity against disease, virus, and other microorganisms, why do we get sick anyway?

It is because we are eating unhealthy foods for taste only that are actually interfering with our natural immunity.

A Healthy Body Has Natural Resistance against Disease

The immune system protects the body against disease or other potentially damaging foreign bodies. When functioning properly, the immune system identifies and attacks a variety of threats, including viruses, bacteria and parasites, while distinguishing them from the body's own healthy tissue.

The Lymphatic system consists of bone marrow, spleen, thymus and lymph nodes.

- Bone marrow produces white blood cells, or leukocytes.
- The spleen - the largest lymphatic organ in the body, contains white blood cells that fight infection or disease.
- The thymus is where T-cells mature. T-cells help destroy infected or cancerous cells.
- Lymph nodes produce and store cells that fight infection and disease.
- Lymphocytes and leukocytes are small white blood cells that play a large role in defending the body against disease.
- The two types of lymphocytes are B-cells, which make antibodies that attack bacteria and toxins, and T-cells, which help destroy infected or cancerous cells.
- Leukocytes are white blood cells that identify and eliminate pathogens .

The first thing you need to give up is white sugar – the highly processed treat we have all grown to love and that has become a major staple in most all meals. It is often added by the diner as a syrup, sprinkles, frostings, or eaten in ice cream, candy, cookies, cakes, and other favorite sweets.

Sugar gives you lots of quick (but short-lived) energy, and gives you a feel-good feeling for a little while. Yet that sugar is attacking your body and will be explained more in this book.

A healthy body tests slightly acidic and is able to fight off infections. One that is overly alkaline is sick and unable to heal as the tissues, organs, skin, blood in the arteries and vessels, and even the brain will start to deteriorate.

However, a system can be TOO acidic. Being too acidic is not suitable for your body. This condition may conceive various symptoms which cause you to suffer from them. You may think you have harmful diseases, and you have a weak immune system, etc. But probably the main reason for all of these is just too acidic. Therefore, you need to check the list of symptoms of being too acidic and start a more alkaline diet.

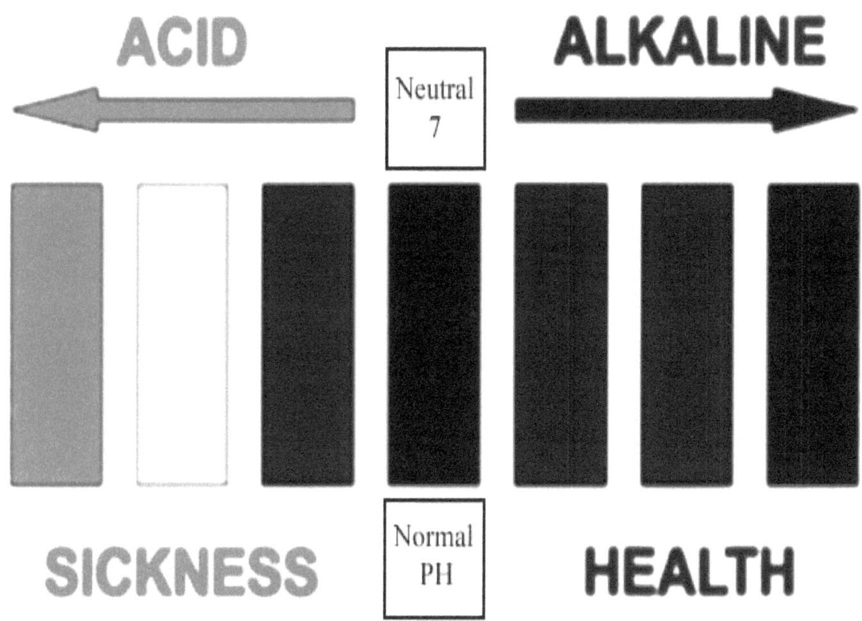

Being too acidic is not suitable for your body. This condition may conceive various symptoms which cause you to suffer from them. You may think you have harmful diseases, and you have a weak immune system, etc. But probably the main reason for all of these is just too acidic. Therefore, you need to check the list of symptoms of being too acidic and may jump into the alkaline diet. Follows is the list of symptoms of being too acidic:

Having Unhealthy Skin

Having unhealthy skin is just one of the symptoms of being too acidic. If your nails are thin and you complain that they break easily, the cosmetics can't help you. Plus, you may have dry skin, and your lips' corners may crack. Again the cosmetics can't solve this. Also, being too acidic cause hair fall, too.

Having Unhealthy Mouth and Teeth

Being too acidic can cause not only sensitive teeth but also losing your teeth. So, you may usually have tooth pain and sensitive gums.

Having Digestive Problems

Lots of people suffer from digestive problems. Being too acidic make digestion harder. So that can cause acid reflux, ulcers, and gastritis. You may have one of the disorders.

Being Joyless and Depressed

If you feel like you're in a depression and if the drugs are useless, try to think about acidic foods. Acidic foods cause having low energy and joyless. Also, you may feel much nervous.

Being Too Acidic Affects Your Whole Body

If you usually consume acidic foods, you may often have headaches, leg cramps, and conjunctivitis because this condition affects not only your metabolism but your eye health too. Having a low body temperature is one of the symptoms, also. If you get infections quickly or if you have a tendency for it, that is because of being too acidic.

How to avoid being too acidic.

The path to an alkaline lifestyle is not difficult. By keeping the ratio of acidic food at around 30% and alkaline diet at approximately 70% will do the trick.. Suggestions follow:

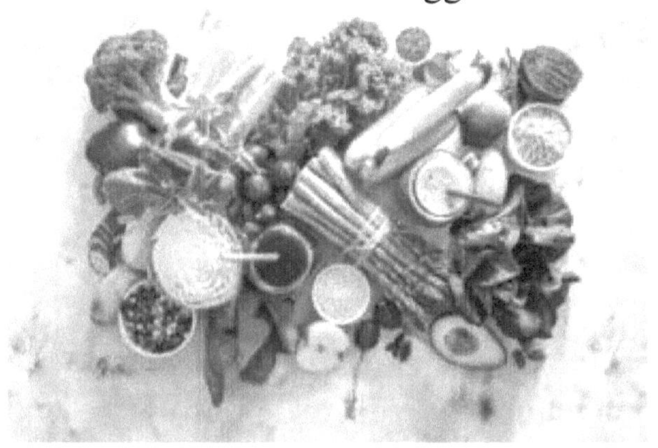

1. Go green

Vegetables, some fruits, seeds, nuts, and roots are naturally alkalizing. Increasing the amount of these in your diet will automatically reduce your consumption of acidic foods like meat or grains. Avocados, beetroot, spinach, kale (if you have access to it it is at the top of the nutrition/calorie chart), cucumber are going to boost your alkalinity.

2. Consume acidic foods mindfully

It is challenging to cut out these naturally addictive foods such as any meat, eggs, processed sugars, flour, and dairy products. However, it is considerably easier to reduce their amount in your daily diet to less than 30%.

3. Limit alcohol consumption

Alcohol may cause different issues in our lives. However, it inevitably causes dietary problems due to very high sugar content. An occasional glass of wine or a few beers enjoying a sports game is acceptable for social benefit. However, alcohol should be consumed responsibly. Otherwise, it makes the body acidic very quickly.

4. Drinking alkaline water

First of all, we have to admit that most of us do not drink enough water. Everyone has to drink 8 to 10 large glasses of water every day, preferably alkaline water. Tap water or bottled water has a pH of up to 7, whereas alkaline water has an average pH of 9. This helps at balancing the alkaline-acid levels in the body.

5. Choose drinks carefully

Caffeine-containing drinks such as coffee and energy drinks usually urges you to consume more sugar. Choosing natural, alkalizing drinks such as herbal teas (peppermint, yerba mate etc..), lemon water and green powder supplements such as green vibrance can help cleanse the digestive system, optimize metabolism and eradicates excess acid.

Lemon water and green powder supplements can help cleanse the digestive system, optimize metabolism and eradicates excess acid.

There is more explanation later on how sugar is made and how the manufacturing process leaves no nutrients.

Seven things you should know about the Coronavirus

This section was written by a registered nurse in 2020.

1. Coronavirus itself isn't new. Just like influenza, coronavirus is a family of respiratory viruses, and there are multiple strains, which have the ability to change over time. Coronavirus is already common in the United States, and has been for years. I have personally cared for patients with this diagnosis.

2. Novel coronavirus, also known as COVID-19, is the strain we're hearing about in the news. It emerged in Wuhan, China at the end of 2019.

3. Symptoms of COVID-19 include fever, cough, and shortness of breath. Just like the flu and common cold, it is spread person to person via respiratory droplets when an infected person coughs or sneezes.

4. According to the World Health Organization, as of February 26, there have been 2,918 confirmed cases of COVID-19 outside of China. 53 of these are in the United States. There have been 44 deaths, none in the United States. Compare this to influenza, which the CDC estimates will infect between 29,000,000 and 41,000,000 people in the United States alone during the 2019-20 season, resulting in 16,000 to 41,000 deaths.

5. "But there's no cure!" You're right. There's no magic pill that cures the flu either. But there is a flu vaccine (that doesn't cause autism) that can protect you from our most common respiratory viruses. Maybe go get one.

6. So, why are we panicking? Frankly, because the media tells us to. Manufacturing a pandemic is a great way to boost ratings, but everything science knows so far about COVID-19 has revealed it to be no more than yet another respiratory virus (and there are thousands).

7. The scariest part of COVID-19 isn't the virus itself, it's the resulting baseless mass paranoia. Hospitals are hoarding supplies, creating shortages of PPE necessary to protect

healthcare workers and patients. Cities are refusing to house and treat sick people who have nowhere else to go. People are using the virus as an excuse for their own social prejudices.

So, what can you do? Turn off the TV and arm yourself with the facts. Stop the spread of false information.

And for Pete's sake, wash your hands.

(Information & statistics obtained directly from the CDC & WHO TV)

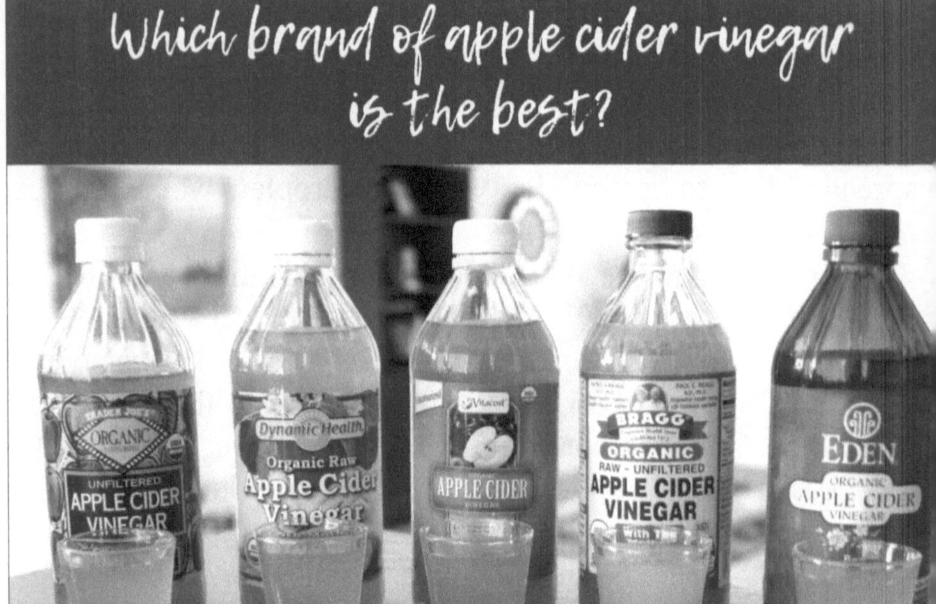

Lots of choices. Apple Cider Vinegar even comes in pills/tablets. Keep in mind that to digest a pill or tablet takes a little longer than drinking the liquid which is absorbed into your blood stream through the stomach much faster to do its work.

Author does not endorse any particular brand. Just make sure it is "Apple Cider Vineger" and NOT "Apple Cider <u>Flavored</u> Vinegar" which is not the same thing.

Benefits of Apple Cider Vinegar

Author's warnings:

1) Apple Cider <u>Flavored</u> vinegar is NOT the same thing as pure Apple Cider Vinegar.

2) <u>White Vinegar</u> is NOT the same as Pure Apple Cider Vinegar. Normally any bottle that lists the contents as "Apple Cider Vinegar" with no other wording IS the right solution.

3) A dose of 1 teaspoon of Apple Cider Vinegar is all that is necessary to correct a temporary PH imbalance and may safely be taken twice a day in water or fruit/vegetable juice. It should not be taken with medication but is quickly digested through the stomach so can be taken ½ hour before or after scheduled medications.

ACV should also not be taken without a liquid to wash it down. When it reaches the stomach acidity it is harmless and does its work along with normal stomach acids to help digest food and absorbed through the circulatory system (blood) to clear out plaque and disable and destroy any virus that are invading your body.

If you drink Apple Cider Vinegar without a cushioning liquid like water or juice, it may irritate your throat and pit your teeth. The stomach can handle acid which it creates on its own to digest your food. Your mouth and throat are easily irritated when coming in direct contact with undiluted Apple Cider Vinegar.

Also DO NOT overindulge in Apple Cider Vinegar. Too much can worsen your Acid/Alkaline imbalance and worsen any conditions you are already dealing with. I know one man who decided to drink a cup of Apple Cider Vinegar even through he had been told to use no more than 1 teaspoon twice a day in water or other liquid. He got a major belly ache that night and realized how dangerous an overdose can be and which can even cause stomach ulcers.

Apple cider vinegar has been around for a long time. Its use dates back thousands of years. It's been used for detoxification, treating pneumonia, and assisting with weight loss. Some claim that the ancient Greek physician Hippocrates used it to cure a host of ailments.

When it comes to weight loss, the apple cider vinegar diet isn't like a lot of the others on the market. All it requires is adding a little bit of apple cider vinegar to your (hopefully) sensible diet. Recommendations vary, but sensible approaches involve either drinking a teaspoon of apple cider vinegar before meals and/or adding apple cider vinegar to meals.

How does Apple Cider Vinegar work?

So how does apple cider vinegar help people lose weight and become resistant to virus infections, common colds, bronchitis, etc? It accelerates the body's ability to break down and derive nutrients from fats and protein efficiently and quickly from the digestive system, which means a faster metabolism and more vitality to fight internal germs and virus looking for a tolerable and accepting host to multiply. A body with a PH imbalance is a welcome place for germs, virus, and other diseases/disorders to multiply.

Both apple cider vinegar and raw apples contain the fiber pectin. There is evidence to suggest that fibers like pectin can increase a person's sense of fullness after they eat it, which lowers their desire to overeat or compulsively snack.

In a 2014 review, researchers found that while there is some evidence that vinegars can help with hyperglycemia (high blood sugar) and obesity, there is no evidence that it positively affects metabolism. However, one 2016 study done on rats showed an improvement in satiation (fullness), cholesterol, and blood sugar after taking apple cider vinegar. This preliminary study indicated that "metabolic disorders caused by a high fat diet are thwarted by taking apple cider vinegar."

What are other benefits of Apple Cider Vinegar?

While vinegar seems to have an acidic quality to it, it actually does just the opposite in your body. "Apple cider vinegar helps the body maintain an alkaline pH, which is widely regarded as anti-cancer and promotes general vitality and wellbeing," says Jansen.

Your body's pH is a measure of your body's acidity and alkalinity. Severe acidity can lead to a number of health problems, like acidosis which affects the kidneys, lungs and resulting kidney stones.

Recent studies support the observation that apple cider vinegar is beneficial for managing post-meal blood sugar levels or spikes. This can be very helpful for people with diabetes. Keeping your alkaline pH balanced is essential for maintaining good health. Severe acidity can lead to a number of health problems, like acidosis and kidney stones.

Apple cider vinegar as a supplement or applied topically can also be good for the skin. When applied topically, it regulates the pH of the skin and has a great effect fighting age spots, acne, and even warts, "It has a detoxifying effect on the liver which will show up in a glowing healthy complexion. Its beneficial bacteria will contribute to healthy skin as well, because our skin is a reflection of what is inside us as well as what is outside us."

Reminder

People who intend to use apple cider vinegar should ensure that it is heavily diluted. Normal dosage is 1 teaspoon of Apple Cider Vinegar diluted with a cup of water, V8 juice or other natural juice is the safest. "Make sure you rinse your mouth with water afterwards," says Jansen.

A teaspoon of Apple Cider Vinegar with a cup of liquid (water, juice) is normally digested and absorbed into the circulatory system (blood) where it does its work eliminating virus, thinning blood clots, and more.

Steps to Achieve a healthy PH-balance

Your body's pH balance, also referred to as its acid-base balance, is the level of acids and bases in your blood at which your body functions best. A normal blood pH level is 7.40 on a scale of 0 to 14, where 0 is the most acidic and 14 is the most basic.

This value can vary slightly in either direction. Fortunately, making your organism more alkaline is simple and is the opposite of acidic environment.

Here are 10 simple natural ways that you can practice every day to alkalize your organism. You will soon gain more everyday energy and vitality:

1) The most important thing is to start your day with a large glass of water with the juice of a freshly-squeezed lemon. Lemons actually have the opposite effect on your body even they may seem acidic. Drink first thing in the morning to flush the system.

2) Another option is to drink one or two glasses of water with organic apple cider vinegar. You should dilute one tablespoons of pure apple cider vinegar in eight ounces of water.

3) Eat a large portion of green salad tossed in lemon juice and quality olive oil. Greens (vegetable or fruit) are among the best sources of alkaline minerals, like calcium. Eat alkaline foods during the day like fruits and vegetables. They sustain the body's pH on a daily basis and keep balance in your organism.

4) Your snack should consist on raw, unsalted almonds. Almonds are full of minerals that are natural alkaline like magnesium and calcium, which actually help to balance out acidity and at the same time to balance blood sugar.

5) Drink almond milk and make yourself a berry smoothie with added green powder like spirulina, or other greens. If

you have choice between almond milk and cow's milk, almond milk is better option.

6) Go for a walk or some other exercise. It's very important to be active. Exercise actually helps move acidic products so your body can better eliminate them.

7) Breathe deeply. Ideally choose a spot that has fresh, oxygen-rich air and go there whenever you can. If you live in a city with tall buildings and lots of automobile traffic, you may need to find a quiet side-street where there would be fresher air not filled with auto exhaust fumes. Continue to drink lots of water on daily basis to flush the system of waste.

8) Do not eat meat every day. If you can skip a few days without meat it will be help get rid of excess acid. Eating meat every day leaves an acid residue behind. On non-meat days you can select vegan or vegetarian entrees to help Alkalize your body!

9) Add more vegetables to your diet. Be careful, potatoes don't count. However, sweet potatoes are good choice but don't make them with butter, use olive oil and Himalayan salt for baking. Peppers, Asparagus, squash, and other vegetables are also great choices.

10) And last but not least: Add more sprouts to your daily diet. They are extremely alkalizing and rich in nutrients and energy-boosting enzymes.

11) Skip desserts loaded with sugar and skip drinking soda. Sugar is one of the worst acidic foods we consume and is our enemy. If you drink just ONE can of soda with sugar, you will actually need more than thirty glasses of neutral water to neutralize the acidity in your body! A person can survive with better health if they omit all pure sugars from their diet.

The Four Sugars

Glucose is the sugar in blood, and **dextrose** is the name given to glucose produced from corn. Biochemically they are identical.

Fructose is the principal sugar in fruit. It raises no issues in fruit because it is accompanied by nutrients and fiber.

Sucrose is table sugar. It is a double sugar, containing one part each of glucose (50%) and fructose (50%), chemically bound together. Enzymes in the intestine quickly and efficiently split sucrose into glucose and fructose, which are absorbed into the body as single sugars.

High Fructose Corn Syrup or HFCS is made from corn starch. It contains roughly equivalent amounts of glucose (45 to 58%) and fructose (42 to 55%). HFCS raises several issues, <u>health</u> and otherwise:

Concerns about High Fructose Corn Syrup

U S Americans (all ages) consume about 60 pounds of sucrose and <u>another 60 pounds of HFCS each year</u>. This is way more than is good for health. Sugars of any kind provide calories but **NO** nutrients.

Increasing evidence suggests that the metabolism of Fructose which differs from that of glucose is associated with abnormalities. This means that it is best to reduce intake of fructose from table sugar as well as HFCS.

There is no reason to study or memorize the following Sugar chart in the next chapter. Basically sugar is a non-food (unless it is part of a healthy fruit) and does little good but causes damage in the human body. You will be more susceptible to colds, flu and other virus infections, diabetes, heart disease, and even kidney failure if you add lots of sugar to your diet..

Table of Sugar Comparisons of Human Tolerance

Sugar	Description	HFI Tolerance
Agave Syrup	From the blue agave cactus. Commonly used in Tex-Mex foods, tequila, margaritas, soft drinks. High in fructose.	Not Tolerated
Aspartame	Sugar substitute known as Equal, NutraSweet, NutraTase. FDA approved. Scientifically studied in depth. Some may be sensitive to headaches.Derived from amino acids.	Tolerated
Acesulfame-K	Sugar substitute known as Sunette, SwissSweet, Sweet-One. Was approved by FDA, but Center for Science in the Public Interest (CSPI) recently questioned safety. Possible carcinogenic.	Tolerated (Questionable safety)
Baker's Sugar	Another name for Bar Sugar, Berry Sugar, Castor/Caster sugar, Ultrafine,Superfine. Sucrose, Finest of all granulated sugar.	Not Tolerated
Bar Sugar	Another name for Baker's Sugar, Berry Sugar, Castor/Caster sugar, Ultrafine, Superfine. Sucrose, Finest of all granulated sugar.	Not Tolerated
Barbados Sugar	British specialty brown sugar with strong molasses flavor.	Not Tolerated
Barley Malt Syrup	From sprouted grains of barley, kiln dried and cooked with water.	Tolerated
Beet Sugar	Sucrose. Same structure as cane sugar, but may produce different product results because of .05 differences in minerals and proteins. More common in Europe than the U.S	Not Tolerated

Berry Sugar	Another name for Baker's Sugar, Bar Sugar, Castor/Caster sugar, Ultrafine, Superfine. Sucrose. Finest of all granulated sugar.	Not Tolerated
Birch Sugar	Sugar alcohol: Xylitol. Trade name; The Ultimate Sweetener. Derived from xylose.	Tolerated depending on purity
Brown Rice Syrup	Made from brown rice. High protein content. Likely contains sucrose.	Not Tolerated
Brown Sugar	Sucrose coated with molasses.¬Ý	Not Tolerated
Cane Sugar	Sucrose. Table sugar.	Not Tolerated
Castor/Caster Sugar	Another name for Baker's Sugar, Bar Sugar, Berry Sugar, Superfine, Ultrafine. Sucrose. Finest of all granulated sugar.	Not Tolerated
Carob Powder	75% sucrose, pluse glucose and fructose. Extract of the carob tree.	Not Tolerated
Chicory	Contains inulin. Used to make fructose syrup.	Not Tolerated
Chinese Rock Sugar	Combination of honey and sugars.	Not Tolerated
Corn Starch	Derived from corn. Composed of straight or branched chains of glucose.	Tolerated
Corn Sugar	Produced from corn starch. Contains glucose and maltose molecules.	Tolerated
Corn Syrup	Glucose and water. Usually produced from cornstarch. The problem is that in making the syrup, it may have either maltose and/or fructose added.	Not Tolerated
Corn Syrup Solids	Dried glucose syrup.	Caution, needs further clarification
Confectioners Sugar	Sucrose. A chemical combination of glucose and fructose.	Not Tolerated

Date Sugar	Made from dried, pulverized dates. Likely contains sucrose.	Not Tolerated
Demerara	Sucrose. Another name for raw sugar. A chemical combination of glucose and fructose.	Not Tolerated
Dextrin	Glucose molecules linked together in chains. Does not break down to pure dextrose.	Tolerated
Dextrose	Single glucose molecule. Simple sugar.	Tolerated
Dextroglucose	Single glucose molecule. Simple sugar.	Tolerated
Dextrose Monohydrat	Pure dextrose.	Tolerated
D-Allose	Simple sugar.Not commonly found in diet.Made of 6 carbons.	Tolerated
D-Altrose	Simple sugar.Not commonly found in diet.Made of 6 carbons.	Tolerated
D-Arabinose	Simple sugar.Not commonly found in diet.Made of 5 carbons.	Tolerated
D-Erythrose	Simple sugar.Not commonly found in diet.Made of 4 carbons.	Tolerated
D-Erythrulose	Simple sugar.Not commonly found in diet.Made of 4 carbons.	Tolerated¬Ý
D-Galactose	Simple sugar.Not commonly found in diet as free galactose.Made of 6 carbons.¬ÝPart of lactose.	Tolerated¬Ý
D-Gulose	Simple sugar.Not commonly found in diet.Made of 6 carbons.	Tolerated
D-Idose	Simple sugar.Not commonly found in diet.Made of 6 carbons.	Tolerated
D-Lyxose	Simple sugar.Not commonly found in diet.Made of 5 carbons.	Tolerated

D-Psicose	Sweetener.¬ÝMay cause diarrhea. Chemically related to fructose.Made of 6 carbons.	Tolerated depending on purity
D-Ribose	Simple sugar.Not commonly found in diet.Made of 5 carbons.	Tolerated
D-Ribulose	Simple sugar.Not commonly found in diet.Made of 5 carbons.	Tolerated
D-Sorbose	Sweetener.May cause diarrhea. Chemically related to fructose.Made of 6 carbons.	Tolerated depending on purity
D-Tagatose	Sweetener.¬ÝMay cause diarrhea. Chemically related to fructose.Made of 6 carbons.	Tolerated depending on purity
D-Talose	Simple sugar.Not commonly found in diet.Made of 6 carbons.	Tolerated
D-Threose	Simple sugar.Not commonly found in diet.Made of 4 carbons.	Tolerated
D-Xylose	Simple sugar.Not commonly found.Made of 5 carbons.	Tolerated
D-Xyulose	Simple sugar.Not commonly found in diet.Made of 5 carbons.	Tolerated
Dulcitol	Naturally occurring sugar alcohol.	Not Tolerated
Erythitol	Sugar alcohol. Related to erythrose.	Tolerated depending on purity
Evaporated Cane Sug	Sucrose. Another name for sugar cane juice.	Not Tolerated
Fructose	Simple sugar of fructose molecules. Sometimes called fruit sugar.Made of 6 carbons.	Not Tolerated
Fruit Juice Sweetene	Derived from grapes, apples or pears, heated to reduce water leaving a sweeter moreconcentrated juice.Almost pure fructose.	Not Tolerated
Gemsugar	Colored sugar made from Thai sugarcane infused with herbs.	Not Tolerated

Glucose	Simple sugar. The chemical sugar structure of blood sugar.Made of 6 carbons.	Tolerated
Glucose Polymers	Chains of glucose molecules.	Tolerated
Glucose Syrups	Produced from starch, corn syrup, corn-syrup solids, starch syrup, and sugar cane syrup. Another name for glucose.	Caution, needs further clarification
Grape Syrup	Pure fructose.	Not Tolerated
Granulated sugar	Table sugar. Sucrose.¬Ý	Not Tolerated
Gur	Another name for Jaggery. 35% sucrose, 15% reducing sugar (mixture of glucose plus fructose). Used in Thai cooking. Made from palm dates or sugar cane juice. Contains molasses.	Not Tolerated
High Fructose Corn S	Enzymetically converted from corn syrup to contain 42% - 90% fructose. Raises triglyceride levels and increases risk of heart disease.	Not Tolerated
High Fructose glucos	Contains fructose.	Not Tolerated
Honey¬Ý	Natural syrup containing about 35% glucose, 40% fructose, 25 % water	Not Tolerated
Hydrogenated Starch	Sugar alcohol of glucose.	Tolerated depending on purity
Invert Sugar	Created by combining sugar syrup with cream of tarter or lemon juice and heating, breaking sucrose down to components glucose and fructose.	Not Tolerated
Isoglucose	Another name for High Fructose Corn Syrup (HFCS).	Not Tolerated
Isomaltose	Linked glucose molecules that rapidly break down to glucose	Tolerated

	in the intestine.	
Jaggery	Made from either evaporating fresh juice of palm trees, or sugar cane juice. 35% sucrose, 15% reducing sugar (mixture of glucose plus fructose). Contains molasses.	Not Tolerated
Lactitol	Sugar alcohol form of lactose.	Tolerated depending on purity
Lactose	Milk sugar, making up 4.5% of cow's milk. Restricted in lactose intolerant.	Tolerated
Levulose	Contains fructose.	Not Tolerated
Litesse	Polydextrose. Nondigestable polysaccharide. Reduced calorie sugar substitute containing sorbitol and glucose.	Not Tolerated
Maltitol	Sugar alcohol form of maltose (glucose).	Tolerated depending on purity
Maltose	Linked glucose molecules that rapidly break down to glucose in the intestine.¬Ý	Tolerated
Maltodextrin	Dextrose. Processed from natural cornstarch.	Tolerated
Mannitol	Sugar alcohol form of mannose.	Tolerated depending on purity
Mannose	Simple sugar.Not commonly found.	Tolerated
Maple Syrup	Mostly sucrose. Contains some invert sugar.	Not Tolerated
Maple Sugar	Mostly sucrose. Contains some invert sugar.	Not Tolerated
Moducal	Glucose chains. A medical food. Consult physician before use.¬Ý	Tolerated

Molasses	By-product of sugar cane with 24% water. Fructose level varies. Three kinds. Light (sweetest), Medium (darker and less sweet), Blackstrap (very dark, slightly sweet with distinctive flavor. Good source of calcium and iron)	Not Tolerated
Molasses Sugar	Dark muscovado sugar with extra molasses.	Not Tolerated
Muscovado Sugar	Another name for Barbados sugar, a brown sugar with strong molasses flavor.	Not Tolerated
Neotame	Sugar substitute. Synthetic aspartame.	Tolerated
Palm Sugar	Used in Thai cooking. Likely contains sucrose.	Not Tolerated
Panella	35% sucrose, 15% reducing sugar (mixture of glucose plus fructose.) Contains molasses.	Not Tolerated
Polincillo¬Ý	Mexican brown sugar. Semi refined and granulated. No molasses added	Not Tolerated
Polycose	Chains of dextrose. Added to foods to increase calories.	Tolerated
Polydextrin	Chains of glucose molecules. Does not break down to pure dextrose.	Tolerated
Polydextrose	Polydextrose is a multi-purpose additive synthesized from dextrose (glucose), plus about 10 percent sorbitol and 1 percent citric acid. It is commonly used as a replacement for sugar, starch, and fat in commercial cakes, candies, dessert mixes, gelatins, frozen desserts, puddings, and salad dressings.¬ÝSorbitol is a sugar alcohol that is related to fructose.	Not Tolerated

Raffinose	A trisaccharide found in grains, legumes and some vegetables. Gas forming.	Tolerance Varies
Rapadura	35% sucrose, 15% reducing sugar (glucose plus fructose). Contains molasses.	Not Tolerated
Raw Sugar	Sucrose. Equal parts glucose and fructose, a chemical combination of glucose and fructose.	Not Tolerated
Reducing Sugar	Referred to as invert sugar (mixture of glucose and fructose).	Not Tolerated
Rock Sugar	Crystallized cane sugar. Sucrose, a combination of glucose and fructose.	Not Tolerated
Saccharin	Sugar substitute. Not as commonly used as in the past. Known as Sweet N' Low, Sugar Twin, Sucryl, Featherweight. FDA approved. More than 6 servings per day may increase bladder cancer risk. (No longer approved for use in Canada)	Tolerated
Saccharose	Sucrose. Equal parts glucose and fructose.	Not Tolerated
Sorbitol	Sugar alcohol. Common in fruits, particularly skin of ripe berries, cherries and plums. Used in sugar free foods. Causes diarrhea. Converted back to fructose.	Not Tolerated
Splenda	A sugar substitute. This is a chemically modified sucrose molecule that cannnot be digested.	Tolerated depending on purity
Stevia	Natural sweetener from a South American plant. 30 % sweeter than sugar. Used extensively in Japan, China, Korea, Israel, Brazil and Paraguay with no side effects reported. Known as Stevioside. Has not been rigorously tested	Not Tolerated

	for safety. No consistent manufacturing regulations.¬Ý	
Sucanat	Sucrose. Another name for raw sugar. Equal parts glucose and fructose. However, read the labels. Some now listed as Sucanat are cane sugar plus blackstrap molasses.	Not Tolerated
Sucralose	Chemical name for Splenda, a sugar substitute. Large molecule not digested.	Tolerated depending on purity
Sucrose	Naturally occurring sugar made from sugar cane or sugar beets. Commonly referred to as sugar and table sugar. Chemical combination of glucose and fructose.	Not Tolerated
Sucrose Syrups	Also known as Refiner's syrup. By product of sugar refining. 15 ¬Æ¬¢ 18% water, 1 part sucrose to two parts invert sugar.	Not Tolerated
Sugar	Common name for sucrose, a chemical combination of glucose and fructose.	Not Tolerated
Sugar Alcohol	May be naturally or synthetically occurring. Causes diarrhea. This is a reduced form of sugar that may be metabolized back to fructose or other sugars depending on the type.	Not Tolerated
Trimoline	Produced from beets. Up to 22 % invert sugar. 28 % sweeter than granulated sugar	Not Tolerated
Turbinado	Another name for raw sugar. Sucrose, a chemical combination of glucose and fructose.	Not Tolerated

Vanilla sugar	Sucrose. Made by burying vanilla beans in cane sugar for weeks. A chemical combination of glucose and fructose.	Not Tolerated
Wasanbon	Grown on an island in the area of Japan from a special variety of sugar cane. A pale beige powder of very pure sugar. Not good for cooking. Melts immediately on the tongue. Very scarce and very expensive.	Not Tolerated
Xylitol	Sugar alcohol. Obtained from fruits and berries. Also from birch trees and known as birch sugar. Causes diarrhea.	Tolerated depending on purity
Xylose	Simple sugar.Not commonly found.¬ÝMade of 5 carbons.	Tolerated

The Best 15 Alkaline Foods on the Planet

1. Spinach

Spinach can eliminate free radicals, improve your memory, and keep your heart strong by being rich in antioxidants. Furthermore, it can stimulate your brain function. It is low in fat and cholesterol, it has vitamins A, C, K, B6, and contains magnesium, potassium, calcium, zinc, iron, and niacin.

2. Lemons

The lemon juice can reduce the risk of stroke, and it can also help treat kidney stones. Another positive side to the lemon is that it helps fight cancer, prevent constipation and high blood pressure. It has vitamins E, A, C, B6, and many important minerals like zinc, calcium, potassium, copper, and riboflavin.

3. Quinoa

It can help with the cholesterol and blood sugar level in your body. It is the food that is the richest in proteins and compared to other grains it has twice the amount of fiber. Moreover, quinoa is rich in manganese, magnesium, riboflavin, lysine and iron.

4. Swiss Chard

The Swiss chard helps with blood sugar, and improves the health of your heart and your blood circulation. It helps the body stay away from viruses, harmful bacteria, and free radicals. Also, it is the best source of alkali from all foods known to us.

5. Buckwheat

This wheat is nothing like the regular one, since it can improve your heart health, prevent diabetes, and boost your energy levels. It keeps your body warm, so it's a perfect meal for the winter's cold days. In addition, buckwheat is a great source of vitamins, iron, and protein.

6. Melon

The melon will clear the toxins from your body and at the same time keep you hydrated. What makes it a top alkaline food is its pH value that is around 8,5. The water content of this fruit is very high, and that is why it is a good example of an alkaline food.

7. Olive oil

Olive oil regulates the blood sugar levels and reduces the risk of heart disease. It is rich in vitamin E, monounsaturated fatty acids, and antioxidants. So, we recommend adding it to your diet.

8. Bananas

If you want to lose weight you better add bananas to your daily diet. This fruit balances the blood sugar levels, protects the heart and improves the digestion. In addition, it is rich in fiber and nutrients like potassium, manganese, B vitamins, and magnesium.

9. Flaxseed

These seeds keep the heart healthy, help control the hot flashes in menopause and reduce inflammations. The flaxseed is considered as a top alkaline food since it is rich in fiber, antioxidants and vitamin E. Therefore, we recommend you use it every day. You can grind the flaxseed and add it to almost any meal.

10. Cauliflower

It boosts the heart health and has anti-inflammatory properties. One serving of this vegetable provides 77 percent of the daily requirement of vitamin C. Moreover, cauliflower is abundant in riboflavin, potassium, magnesium, vitamin K, thiamin, and manganese.

11. Avocados

Avocados help the absorption of nutrients from vegetables and fruits, control the levels of cholesterol and make your heart stronger. You can reap the benefits of this super-food by consuming even a bowl of guacamole. What's more, the avocado contains fiber, nutrients, and monounsaturated fatty acids.

12. Grapes

They help reduce anxiety and hypertension. This fruit reduces the risk of lung, prostate, colon, esophageal, pancreatic, endometrial, and mouth cancer, due to its polyphenols (antioxidants).

13. Carrots

Carrots improve your thought process and your eyesight due to their beta-carotene content (a group of pigments) which protect you against free radical damage. They are high in vitamin K, C, A, B8, iron, potassium, and fiber.

14. Broccoli

This vegetable improves the blood circulation due to its high amounts of iron. It keeps the heart healthy, improves the health of bones, and reduces the levels of cholesterol. What's more, broccoli is also a powerful antioxidant which helps fight cancer. It is rich in copper, fiber, potassium and vitamin K, B6, C, and E.

15. Berries

Berries improve the skin and are good food to slow down the aging process. They help with chronic health disorders, and keep a sharp memory as you grow old.

Suggested Shopping List:

Proteins: Low-fat milk, eggs, tinned tuna or sardines, lean beef, chicken or soya mince, chicken portions or breasts

Plant proteins: All types of dry beans, soya beans, lentils and chickpeas

Healthy starch: Rolled oats, brown rice, pearled barley or seeded health bread

Fruit and vegetables: Seasonal fruit, bananas, lemons, tinned and fresh tomatoes, cucumber, carrots, onions, gem squash, cabbage, butternut and spinach

Fats: Light mayonnaise, peanut butter, olive or canola oil

Other: Herbs and spices, salt and pepper, tea and coffee

Where Our Nutrients Come From

The most essential mineral elements of the body composition, in order of their apparent importance, are iodine, copper, calcium, phosphorus, manganese, sodium, potassium, magnesium, chlorine, and sulfur. All but the first of these, iodine, which is a native of the sea, have their source in the soil.

We would naturally suppose that when we eat products of the soil we should secure an ample supply of them. That is whant Nature intended. But Nature did not foresee that man would remove the trees and other growth, allowing the rains to erode the soil, leaching out the essential minerals and, my means of our creeks and rivers, carrying them down to the sea. The result has been mineral-starved soils, in turn producing mineral-starved foods. the obvious result is that humans, how depend upon these mineral-starved foods for our supply of minerals, are literally starving in the midst of plenty.

It is easy to know when one is hunger for sweets, starches, or fats. The body sends out distress signals almost immediately and, if we are in normal health, our appetite tells us what is needed.

Once we learn to know them, the signs of mineral hunger are quite as definite and the results, if our body's SOS it long ignored, are far more serious.

There have developed within the last few generations, especially here in the United States, where food is most abundant and the average person eats most generously a whole series of deficiency diseases. It is recognized that each of these diseases is due to a lack of vital elements in t he diet, and the essentials most often lacking are the essential minerals. The thyroid requires iodine. The parathyroid requires cobalt and nickel. The adrenal glands require magnesium. The pancreas requires cobalt and nickel. The anterior pituitary gland needs manganese. The posterior pituitary needs chlorine. The gonads require iron.

Iron enters directly into the construction of the hemoglobin of red corpuscles, which are the oxygen carriers of our blood. Anemia is a deficiency disease which may develop if there is an insufficient supply of iron in the blood. Unfortunately the human body cannot store up much iron, to it is necessary to replenish the supply regularly.

As our soils become more impoverished, the seas become richer in those minerals. However, we find an ocean plant whose botanical name is Macrocystis pyrifera and which is commonly called *kelp*. It is often referred to as a sea vegetable and serves well as a food supplement.

Kelp grows in great abundance off the California coast. It flourishes best at a depth of six to ten fathoms and is found only where the ocean bottom is rocky. It has no roots but is anchored to the rocks by tough ropelike cables and derives its nourishment entirely from the water. It is one of the largest plants in existence, often growing as much as fifty feet in a single year. Each plant consists of a trunk or stem, lined on either side with large single lanceolate leaves. The leaves occur in files of six or eight or more, the files alternating, each leaf supported by a buoy or floater at its point of contact with the trunk of the plant. Each leaf is finely but irregularly corrugated, is bordered with a single row of short, soft spines, and is olive brown in color.

Biochemistry teaches us that plants are the only organisms that can manufacture food, and that the essential food elements man receives from the flesh of animals come originally from plants. As every raw material essential for plant life is right at hand, the seaweeds such as kelp are naturally rich in the food elements required by man and other forms of animal life. The minerals it absorbs from the water in such abundance are present in an organic colloidal state, readily usable, and directly transferrable to the human body.

The Importance of Iodine

Folk medicine in Vermont is interested in three R's –
Resistance, Repair, and Recovery. First the individual asks
himself whether his resistance to disease is as it should be. Next,
is he able to repair tissue injury due to accident should it occur?
Finally, if sickness should occur, is his body able to bring about
recovery?

Iodine is necessary for the thyroid gland's proper performance
of its work. All the blood in the body passes through the thyroid
gland every 17 minutes. Strong, virulent germs are rendered
weaker during their passage through the thyroid gland. With
each 17 minutes that rolls around they are made still weaker until
finally they are killed *if* the gland has it normal supply of Iodine.

This gland also rebuilds energy and endurance in the
individual. Iodine also relieves nervous tension. When nervous
tension runs high there is irritability and difficulty in sleeping
well at night. The body is continually on a combat basis,
organized for fight and flight. Iodine can relax the body and
enable it to organize for peace and quiet. Iodine also relates to
clear thinking.

One cause for the thyroid to lose Iodine is sodium chloride or
"Table Salt".

Here are three ways to bring up the iodine content when
needed:

1. Eat foods that particularly high in iodine. Radishes,
   asparagus, carrots, tomatoes, spinach, rhubarb, potatoes,
   peas, strawberries, mushrooms, lettuce, bananas,
   cabbage, egg yolk and onions contain iodine.
2. You may also paint a small area of the body with tincture
   of Iodine which is then absorbed through the skin.
3. Preparations known to be rich in iodine include Cod-
   liver oil, Lugol's solution of iodine, and kelp tablets.

One executive's answer to keep his blood on the thin, free-flowing side is by omitting wheat foods, wheat cereals, white sugar, and citrus fruits and fruit juices. The reasoning is because in most people, those foods change the normal acid reaction of the urine to alkaline – a signal that the blood is thicker than it should be causing more work on the heart.

Therefore the man omits and replaces the unwise foods with rye and corn foods and cereals. Instead of white sugar he uses honey. In place of citrus foods and juices, he may use apple, grape, or cranberry juice.

At lunchtime he takes two teaspoonfuls of apple cider vinegar and two teaspoonfuls of honey in a glass of water. In this way he obtains acid taken up from the soil by fruit, berries, edible leaves, and roots, and the energy from the sun which exists in honey. This is a prime pick-up drink.

Observations have been made in the use of Corn oils such as Mazola Oil. One tablespoon of corn oil at one or all three meals each day had been helpful in hay fever, asthma, and migraine, because it helps in keeping the urine on the acid side. Corn oil is of value in shifting the body chemistry from alkaline to acid.

If the margins of the eyelids are scaly and granulated, one tablespoonful of corn oil by mouth at breakfast, and again at the evening meal, will, within one month's time, generally cure the condition. The same treatment for eczema is to remove scales leaving the skin soft and pliable.

Feel free to order a copy of the book "Vermont Folk Medicine"by D. C. Jarvis, M.D. with the subtitle: "A famous doctor's guide to folk medicine practices of Vermont – the nature secrets of honey, apple cider vinegar, and foods for health." Much of the 191 page book also includes tips for livestock care.

These tips may very well protect all of us from the threat of the coronavirus currently assaulting the northern hemisphere. March 5, 2020.

About the Author

Marlys J. Waters was born and raised on a farm near Nemaha, Iowa. After graduating from Crestland Community School (Early and Nemaha) in 1963, she attended Iowa State University and Drake University, and worked thirty years in the Des Moines area.

Marlys returned to her hometown of Nemaha in 1993 to care for her parents where she started "Power of the Pen Publishing. She also writes books and compiles music books for resale.

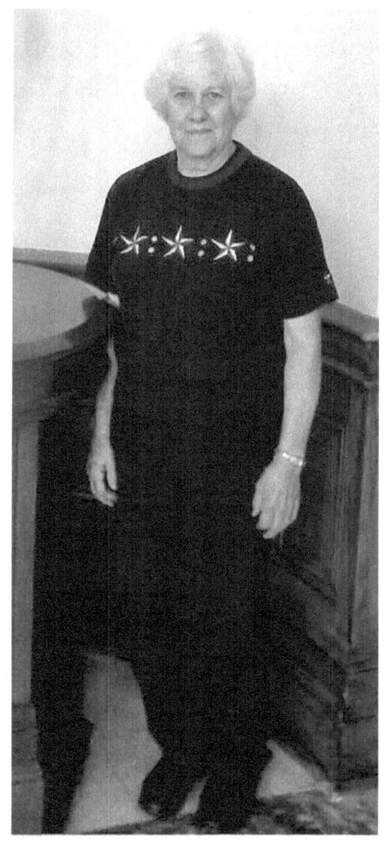

Note: Author Marlys J. Waters gave up common sugar and candy at age 50, and all highly processed sugars at age 65. She lost 50 pounds, and has not needed a doctor's care for over 25 years – no colds, no flu, no coughing, and has retained an active lifestyle at age 74.

She can still walk long distances with no dizzy spells, light knee pain that disappears when resting, and no skin disorders.

Marlys also uses a serving of spinach (cooked, canned, or raw) daily from a tip she learned when she was working full time and taking college classes in her 30s. She had read that spinach would help keep away infections and virus, and would also revitalize her system so she would require less sleep and have more time for work and studies.

She is now sharing her tips on good health to assist others who are struggling with disorders that the doctors are unable to understand and to correct.